For someone who needs a litt [barcode: D1577888] when caring for an older adu you a great perspective on how important it is not to lose yourself in the face of such a daunting disease. Thank you, Patty, for the blessing of this book.

—Terri Lee RN,
Certified Gerontology Specialist

This book is refreshing and uniquely practical for patients and families trying to navigate the complexities of the aging process. In my cardiology practice I regularly deal with older patients whose cardiac and cognitive problems interact and complicate their care. Addressing these concerns with patients and their family members openly and honestly improves care and patient outcomes immensely. I am grateful to have this incredible resource to recommend for anyone who needs help in dealing with family members and the process of aging.

—Dr John Norris MD
Cardiologist

My wife and I both had mothers who struggled with dementia, and this disease produced some of the most painful and confusing days of our lives. Patty Green has written *In Case I Forget* as if she was describing our mothers. We didn't have a clue, we had never experienced anything like this before – we *needed* this book! It is one of the most useful, practical, beautiful books on what to do and how to understand what is happening with our loved ones. AND, Patty helps us prepare for the future. I would highly recommend *In Case I Forget.* Read it, talk about it – let Patty Green help you through the maze of dementia.

—Mark Worley, M.A.
Vice President for Advancement,
Dallas Christian College

I have spent over 25 years in Senior Living in various leadership positions. I feel that it takes a special person to want to work in senior living and it takes an extra special person to excel at caring for those with dementia. Patty is a shining example of one of these extra special people. "In Case I Forget" is a great guide for those facing a diagnosis of dementia. Patty's personal insights and positive outlook provide hope and encouragement when confronting the confusing issues that come with dementia.

—Brian Lane
Director K2M Design Inc

"I remember Dec. 19, 2009 like it was yesterday. That's the day my sweet father passed away from the horrible nightmare that is Lewy Body Dementia. I wouldn't wish that journey on my worst enemy, let alone someone I love. That's been almost a decade now and not a day goes by when I don't think about what dad went through. Which is why I believe Patty Green's book "In Case I Forget" will be a huge encouragement to those families whose loved ones are suffering from the difficult journey of dementia. Her vast experience and insight will prove invaluable to anyone who decides to turn the pages of this helpful and thought provoking book. I love the way Patty uses scripture and story to minister to those of us who have had family members drift down the long, confusing road of dementia. I hope you read this book and I hope it becomes a tremendous help as you care for those you deeply love."

—Drew Sherman, Lead Pastor,
Compass Christian Church DFW

Dementia is a horrible disease that affects not only the patient, but their families as well. Rarely do you come across someone that really "gets" it, and the book "In Case I Forget" demonstrates that Patty Green is one of the few that does. It is immensely practical and reflects Patty's compassionate heart for those suffering with this devastating diagnosis. It offers hope and paints a clear picture of the confusion that is associated with dementia. Thank you for sharing your wisdom and experience as we approach this season of life with our parents and loved ones.

—Matthew LaGrange PhD
Founder & Executive Director
His Story Coaching & Counseling

In Case I Forget

PATTY GREEN CTRS, CDP

In Case I Forget

3 Steps to Take Before Your Memory Unravels

More than 5 million people are living with Alzheimer's disease or other types of dementia and most of us know someone who has it. There is no cure. In most cases, there is no answer to what causes these diseases.

- What if it happens to me?
- If my parent or grandparent had it, what are the chances I will get it?
- Besides a healthy diet high in omega 3 fats and regular exercise - can I prepare?

Based on more than twenty years of experience working with people with dementia, I have written this book to help you and the people you love understand what dementia is and take the 3 practical steps while you can still think clearly to navigate the potential devastation of these diseases.

by Patty Green

Contents

Foreword

First, I pray you will never need this book. I pray a cure is found for dementia before another person needs to think about it as a possibility, much less plan for it, just *in case I forget.*

But…

You don't know what you don't know. And the problem is, there is a chance—a good chance—you won't remember what you need to know without taking action in advance.

When we are younger we call the process "growing up." Once we are adults we are still growing and learning - until we're not. We don't really think about the process of thinking, of how we use our brains, until we see someone we love begin to struggle with it. We may tie a string around a finger to remind us not to forget something and then, seemingly without warning, we develop dementia, and the "growing up" process starts reversing. Inch by inch.

It is so hard to understand this unwelcome disease taking up residence in our minds. I like to try to garden. The idea of fresh herbs and vegetables growing in my back yard is so appealing, and when a friend gave me some wild mint to add I was excited. It smelled amazing and was good in my tea, but in a matter of weeks the stuff took over! I didn't know I needed to pay attention to it. Our minds can be compared to my garden. You've planted wonderful nourishing vegetables of knowledge and maturity, beautiful flowers of precious relationships, but then there is some wild mint, those little forgetful moments, and before you know it, the stuff takes over your whole garden. But there is hope if you start to weed and pay attention your garden! Your garden may not be what you planned, but it can still be worthwhile and valuable.

I am a Certified Therapeutic Recreation Specialist, a Certified Dementia Practitioner, and a Memory Care Director. When a person needs Memory Care, the people who have the hardest time are the loved ones who have to watch dementia steal away the person they love. The person with dementia isn't affected as much, at least in the later stages because they are just coping as they always have - based on who they are.

I have worked in long term care and dementia care since 1995, and through the years I have met and loved some amazing people. People with faith, people with honor, people with humor, people with sadness. Everyone with a unique and wonderful story. These amazing stories have affected me deeply. Their impact has been profound, lasting and has helped me to understand more of what I need to know - *in case I forget*. I never knew the story of who they were before they arrived. I would tell family members, "I didn't know them before the disease, and I love them like they are." I figured out the histories and stories of the people I've cared for in the midst of them losing themselves. I discovered what brought them comfort, by trying to comfort them, I discovered what made them laugh by laughing with them, and I discovered their fears by dealing with the behavior the fears brought. Knowing more of each person's story at the beginning could help me better care for them as the disease progresses.

One night I had hired Robin, an entertainer versed in old favorites, to sing to our care home residents. If you've ever tried to hold the attention of a group of your peers then, you might imagine, performing for a group of eighty to ninety year olds with various levels of alertness could be challenging. Everyone loved Robin as he poured out his heart to the residents and explained some of the history of the old familiar favorites he shared. He built a great connection with them. Robin's joy was evident while singing wonderful old songs that many knew and sang along with. Songs like "Five Foot Two" and "Let Me Call You Sweetheart." Robin had awakened their hearts, and then he began to sing the beautiful love song, "Always" by Irving Berlin. Part of the lyric is "I'll be loving you always, with a love that's true always. Not for just an hour, not for just a day, not for just a year, but always." Betty sat in the front row in her wheelchair. She was tired from her therapy sessions that day, and her silver hair was a little disheveled, but she had looked forward to the evening program. Betty started crying softly at first. Then she was weeping, you could even call it *ugly crying*. She said her heart was breaking. She was howling. We helped her out of the room and were finally able to distract her and comfort her, but we still couldn't understand what had triggered the episode. In my experience, those old songs usually have wonderful memories from younger years for people, and they leave feeling great. But the opposite was true for Betty as her pain was evident in her tears.

Her husband visited later, and we told him about Betty's encounter with this song and how it caused a flow of tears and emotions. He hung his head for a moment, took a deep breath and began to explain: "You see," he said, "'Always' was our song. And 40 years ago I made a terrible mistake. It's hard to even face today—I was unfaithful to her. Since then she couldn't listen to that song without it breaking her heart."

Obviously she had forgiven him, and they had gone on to a long enduring marriage. But we didn't know what we didn't know. Part of caring for people with dementia is getting to know what "triggers" might cause difficult behaviors. Some behaviors are emotional, like Betty's, while others can have strong physical reactions such as hitting others or screaming. If we had known that in her dementia the song would trigger such a heart-wrenching memory for Betty, we could have avoided causing her to re-live that pain by simply asking Robin not to sing that song. If Betty had been widowed, and her husband wasn't there to explain, would her kids have known?— probably not!

Think about Betty's story for a moment. Think about misunderstood behaviors of someone you know who has dementia. This is where the journey begins. What you don't know, what those who will need to care for you don't know, is why I am writing this book. Our life's journey compiled in stories hold the key to our own care journey should **we** develop dementia. ALL the stories of our lives – the good, the bad, the ugly and the joyful – are what give the texture and flavor to our moments and memories. From experience, observation and research, make no mistake about it, the greatest burden of this disease falls to the caregivers.

Giving the potential caregivers in our lives, those people we love dearly, a roadmap is the most important thing you can do. A roadmap reflecting how this journey might unfold and provide answers at each significant age about who we are and how we like life to be. If we can be proactive and provide our stories - *in case we forget* - then maybe our journey can be easier for the ones we leave behind.

We all grow old. There is no getting around it. We don't get to choose how we age. We don't know how it will unfold or how our bodies and minds will be affected by the aging process. As we age, we are still the same person we have always been. Trapped in aging bodies, true, but our spirits are eternal. Our spirits know our own stories, even when we can't tell them anymore ourselves. It is so important to share our stories.

God ordains family relationships, and, though older people can feel they are a burden, our parents have invested in us, their family. They helped us to form values and personalities - quirks and all. Our parents want their families to be proud of them. They want to be remembered and valued. They had influence that shows up in the lives of those who shared their journey. *And so will we when we are their age.* We will want to know that someone remembers us as valuable.

Proverbs 17:6 says, "Children's children are a crown to the aged, and parents are the pride of their children."

If our life path leads us on a journey through dementia, and we have trouble remembering, its good to know this truth from scripture. When we don't remember – God does.

1 Chronicles 16:15 tells us, "He remembers his covenant forever, the promise he made, for a thousand generations."

With the writing of this book I want to honor God who never forgets.

Special Thanks to: God my Father who directs my path and urged me to share what He taught me about this disease and how to navigate it. To my parents Perry & Harriet Lyson and the legacy of love and faith and family I have because of them, my cousin Jim Akers without whose encouragement and insights I would have never actually written this book, my daughter Jessi Rueter who is an excellent word-smith and good friend, my husband Rich who always supports me, and other friends who have helped and encouraged me. To all the people and their families I've known, who have lived and died with this disease, and let me know parts of their stories.

CHAPTER 1

Introduction

In my Memory Care neighborhood everyday is different but the experiences that family members or other visitors share have a few common emotions. Fear. Anxiety. Sadness. Disbelief that this is now reality. For example; You may walk into the memory care neighborhood of the nursing home to see your grandma. It's been a while. You hope she recognizes you. Several people are sitting out at the dining tables. A couple are looking through magazines on the table, some are asleep in their wheelchairs. You don't know any of these folks, you're just there to see Grandma. She's 89 years old. Walking down the hall toward her room there are a variety of sounds: an alarm is going off; someone is moaning; one woman is jabbering incoherently. The smells are equally varied. You smell smells you are unfamiliar with, and there is the chemical smell of cleaning supplies. The place looks clean. Finally you arrive at her room and knock loudly as you enter. "Grandma?" The tiny lady in the wheelchair looks up at you and smiles; she calls you by your Mom's name. "No Grandma, its me - your granddaughter." She looks at you with a question in her eyes. "I think I know my own daughter when I see her! Now, sit right here and tell me how school is going." You do as you're told and sit on her bed, as you try once again to tell her your name and that she is your grandma. She starts to get mad at you, so you change the subject and ask if she'd like you to take her on a wheelchair ride. The rest of the visit goes okay. She never seems to realize who you are and continues to call you by your Mom's name.

Your mind is racing all over as you leave her room. You are caught between the pain of not being remembered and grasping the fondest memories of grandma. All the sights sounds and smells you noticed on your way are being pushed aside and you are overcome with memories of your grandma and how lively she was when she baked bread every day with her favorite country music on the radio. How as a former schoolteacher she always found time to read to you while sitting on her lap. Her favorite fairytale "The Billy Goats Gruff." The joy you felt when the mail man brought the gift of a special quilt made just for you that you still treasure.

You miss her. You sit in your car and pause for a minute. There is so much to digest from this visit You are amazed that she doesn't have those memories of you anymore. It makes you sad. It is natural now for you to wonder if your Mom is going to end up like her Mom. You wonder if <u>you</u> are going to end up that way…

I remember watching my grandpa, my dad's dad. He was always so full of fun. So strong. He had worked for the railroad all his life and raised twelve kids in the harsh climate of North Dakota during the forties and fifties. He loved us grandkids so much, and, even though I didn't see him much more than on our annual trip to North Dakota, he always hugged me and would give a little "whoo!" when I kissed him. He'd chuckle at my jumpy reaction to that and smile at me. He helped me learn how to sketch horses when I was in my "horse craze" around ten years old. We visited my grandparents once when I was a teenager, and I remember when grandpa called my Dad by his brother's name. "Clarence, don't you think its time we got those horses in?" We didn't have any horses. I looked at Dad and asked, "Who's Clarence?" Dad's eyes were sad when he answered and said, "He was his brother. He thinks I'm his brother." As his "hardening of the arteries" (as many called dementia at the time) advanced and got worse, Grandma had to put him in a home. When our family went to visit Grandma, she didn't want any of us kids to go see Grandpa. "Just remember him like he was," she'd say. But I went - for my dad. Grandpa was strapped into his wheelchair with sheets "so he wouldn't hurt himself." It was hard on my Dad—really hard. But he never really talked about it. Was he wondering if it was hereditary? Did he ever think he might be looking in the mirror when he saw his dad? Many families of people suffering from this disease have these questions.

Time can distance you quickly from confronting the realities of dementia. But it never really goes away. It lingers in the back of your mind and you worry that it will come again to visit. So years later when my mom called and said, "Your Dad and I just returned from a trip to the neurologist", I immediately sat down. "The doctor says Dad's got dead spots in his brain. No way to tell if they are new, from little strokes, or if they are old injuries. He also says he has Alzheimer's disease." My mind immediately recalled the last time I saw Grandpa in the nursing home. That can't happen to Dad. But it did.

What if it happens to me?
How can I prepare?
Who will provide my care?
How can I know where to go for help?
Can I afford the care I may need?
How will it affect my family?

My friend Luci is a social worker in the long term care industry. She assists people with nursing home placements, setting up home health and hospice care when needed.

Her Mom has been diagnosed with dementia. She lives ten hours away. Her Dad is healthy and his brain works. She knows what Alzheimer's disease does. Luci works with people who have it everyday. She is busy with three kids and a husband, and a demanding emotional job. Her brother lives close to her parents and is looking in on them regularly. Recently Luci returned home to attend a funeral of a family friend. She noticed her mom hadn't had her finger or toenails cared for in quite some time. Same with her hair. It was a wild mess. So her mom was excited when Luci told her she was going to the spa for hair and nails. Her Mom enjoyed every minute of it and looked so much better afterwards. The next morning, she greeted Luci with a "Hi! When did you get here?" She tried not to cry. Her Mom had forgotten every moment of their lovely spa day.

Luci's mom and dad owned a business, and now her Mom hides things she thinks are valuable. Then of course she forgets. Her Dad is frustrated and exhausted.

Finally over the holidays, Luci was able to have a frank discussion with her dad about how she can help. All he needs, he says, is to talk to Luci every day. So someone will know the day he's had. It breaks her heart, but at least now she feels like she can help in some small way. What if this happens to Luci? How will her family cope if she ends up like her mom? Even with all her experience in assisting others to navigate the disease, it feels very different when it hits home and is personal. She has to deal with the same questions as every family who are victims of this disease. It doesn't really help emotionally, to suspect what is coming.

No one knows the cause. There is no known cure. It touches us in unpredictable ways. There are always more questions than answers. It is the nature of dementia—a disease of the aged that touches every generation of the family it affects. Today in spite of all the medical advancements and research, no one knows the cause and the search for a cure provides limited hope. The reality of this insidious disease is it touches us in unpredictable ways. Everyone has questions and wonders where to turn for answers. That is why I am writing this book - to address the big "WHAT IF?" that anyone who has a loved one with dementia has in the back of his mind. What if that happens to me? Well, it might.

Even though there have been many advances in treatment and early detection, once a person has dementia they must learn to live with it. So let's prepare for the "what if" – in case we forget.

Teach us to number our days aright, that we may gain a heart of wisdom. Psalm90:12

Preparation begins with understanding the general and predictable progression of the disease and how it affects cognition. This becomes the foundation for developing a personalized, three-step plan of care… to help our loved ones navigate the changes this disease might put us through.

What if we don't let this disease steal everything from us by planning ahead?

First let's try to better understand what we may face - *just in case* - we develop dementia.

CHAPTER 2

What Dementia Is and Is Not

Job 12:12
*Is not wisdom found among the **aged**? Does not long life bring understanding?*

Normal Aging – Don't Freak Out

Everyone ages. There are no free passes.

Everyone gets older and people often freak out because they don't understand what normal aging looks like. People can feel like they are unraveling. Normal aging includes the wisdom of long life; the wisdom may just be slower. Don't freak out if it seems too slow.

There is a joke about normal aging that I love:

A pastor goes to visit an elderly lady from his church. "Gladys," he says, "you are getting older, and it is time to think about the hereafter." Gladys pauses and starts to laugh, slapping her knee. "Oh Pastor, I do that all the time! I walk into the kitchen and stand there asking myself 'Now what was I here after?'" This joke is humorous because we can all relate to it. We have all had the experience of forgetting what we intended to do.

Every time my mom goes to get a physical, the doctor gives her a little memory test. She hates it. For the same reason you are likely to hate it. She says it makes her feel dumb. It makes her feel like she can't think well or fast enough, and after it is over and the pressure is off, she thinks of things she should have said. But it is a really good test. Everyone should take it. Take it every year. It's really tough. Ready? Here we go…

Name as many animals as you can in one minute. Have someone make a count for you. One hash mark for each member of the animal kingdom. If you repeat one put a circle. If you say dog twice, one is a circle, but if you say basset hound and cocker spaniel you get a hash mark for each. Ready? Go!

Write down how many you got this year. This is your base line. The diagnostic tests say that if you can name 21 or more your cognition is probably fine. (I know everyone wants to know how many they have to get to be "normal!") If you can only name 15 or less you may have some cognitive impairment. Save your baseline score with your important documents. Check it against how well you do next year.

Why should we play the animal count game?

Just in case.

So we won't freak out.

Face it; we are all scared of what we don't know. The fear is real. When we don't understand what *could* happen we can never be ready if it does. So, what is normal?

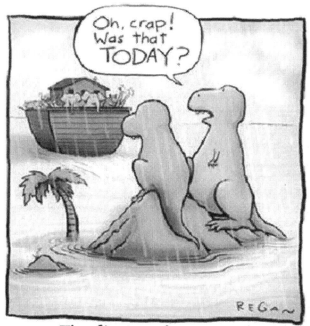

The first senior moment.

Normal Aging includes slower cognitive functioning and some forgetfulness. Normal aging forgetfulness is marked by easily remembering. Think of walking into a room to get something but forgetting what. When you walk back to where you started you get the "oh yeah" moment and retrieve what you started to get. Normal. (Like the joke I shared earlier)

Dementia is more like when you put your remote in the freezer and are convinced someone stole it because you can't find it. (This is a true story. A son lived next door to his Mom and she would always call him because she was certain someone was breaking into her house. She could not follow the logic about why someone would steal her remote and nothing else.)

The most common sign of Alzheimer's is memory loss, especially of recently learned things, *but* forgetting things and remembering them later is completely normal.

- It is normal to occasionally forget what day of the week it is and have to really think about it. However, losing track of the season, such as thinking it is Christmas because your going to church with your family but it is really Easter, is different. This big gap in reality could be an indicator of dementia. This could be difficult to explain, and a hard mistake to cover.
- It is normal to occasionally not be able to come up with the word you need to describe or talk about something. It could indicate dementia if you are repeating the story you just told to the same people or are having difficulty following a conversation.
- It is normal to occasionally need help to work your smart phone or TV, but it could indicate some dementia if you don't remember the rules to a familiar game, or how to get to a familiar place.
- It is normal if you occasionally miss a bill payment, but make it up after you realize it. Dementia could be indicated if you give large donations to telemarketers or buy unneeded items from a home shopping network when you have a fixed income.

As we get older there are lots of things to worry about. Aging is not for the faint of heart! These are some simple scenario examples of experiences many older people could have. People who are dealing with some forgetfulness either find ways to help themselves remember, such as carrying a small note pad and writing down things you don't want to forget, or they can get very good a "covering". They laugh things off and make a joke of it, or try to insinuate they didn't hear correctly. If there is truly a problem, it will become apparent. The point is - don't freak out. Know yourself. Learn. Be prepared for the "what if" - in case you forget.

Types of Dementia

Not all dementia is the same. So, what might we be preparing for?

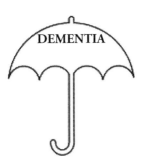

Dementia is the umbrella term for an estimated 110 different types of brain malfunctions. Dementia is defined as a *chronic or persistent disorder of the mental processes caused by brain disease or injury and marked by memory disorders, personality changes, and impaired*

reasoning. Think of cancer – there are so many types of cancer, it is important to understand what type so you can receive the proper treatment. Also, think of having a fever, the fever itself is not the disease, but a symptom of an infection, such as strep throat, or an ear infection or the flu. Similarly dementia is a symptom of something not right in the brain and thinking process.

How is Alzheimer's disease and other dementia diagnosed?

- Medical & Social History
- Mental Status Examination
- Physical Exam
- Neurological Exam: To evaluate for brain disorders other than Alzheimer's
- Lab Tests: To rule out infections, evaluate for vitamin deficiencies, etc.
- Brain Scan: To rule out a tumor or evidence of stroke
- Psychological Evaluation: To evaluate for depression or other mental illness

Like cancer - there are many types: Alzheimer's disease, vascular dementias, lewy body dementias, fronto-temporal lobe dementias, white matter disease, genetic syndrome, infections, and dementias induced by alcohol or drugs, just to name a few. Listed below are descriptions of a few of the most common types.

ALZHEIMER'S DISEASE

Alzheimer's disease is the most common type of dementia. Dr. Alois Alzheimer first identified the disease in 1906. He described the two hallmarks of the disease: "plaques," which are numerous tiny, dense deposits scattered throughout the brain that become toxic to brain cells at excessive levels, and "tangles," which interfere with vital processes, eventually choking off the living cells. When brain cells degenerate and die, the brain markedly shrinks in some regions. I think of the plaque like the plaque that builds up on our teeth - when we go to the dentist for a cleaning, the hygienist often has to work at scraping it off. There is no way to clean that off our brains, so it just keeps building up. As for the tangles, I think about Spiderman's webs. Once they are in one place, they are strong and really gum up the works. This is just how I picture it; the chemistry is more complicated, of course. If you really want to check out the science, there is lots of research. The only fool-proof way to diagnose correctly is during an autopsy after death.

What symptoms are usually present?

- Loss of new information
- Recent memory worsens
- Problems with word finding
- Misspeaking
- More impulsive and indecisive
- Getting lost
- Noticeable changes every 6-12 months
- Typically lasts 8-12 years

VASCULAR DEMENTIA

Vascular dementia is the second most common form of dementia after Alzheimer's disease. Vascular dementia, also called multi-infarct dementia, occurs when the cells in the brain are deprived of oxygen. Although vascular dementia is caused by problems with blood flow to the brain, this blood flow problem can develop in different ways. Stroke is a common cause. Strokes can be large or small, and can have a cumulative effect, which means each stroke adds to the problem. Strokes can affect how a person can walk, and cause weakness in an arm or leg, slurred speech or emotional outbursts, depending on where in the brain it occurs. The difficulties the person has depend on the part of the brain that did not get the oxygen due to the stroke. Another brain injury that affects the brain in a similar way to a stroke is a concussion. Concussions in one's younger years can result in a "dead spot" in the brain. Younger brains usually find ways to work around these spots, but the effect can also be cumulative. The movie starring Will Smith called *Concussion* is a powerful telling of what brain injuries of this sort can do. Vascular dementia usually comes on suddenly. Difficulties may happen in steps. Sometimes, the person's abilities may deteriorate for a while and then stand still for a time. Then, they may deteriorate again. The cognitive symptoms, the ability to think, may change, affecting some areas of the brain more or less than others (e.g., the areas that control language, vision or memory). Urinary difficulties (difficulty going to the bathroom) are common in people who have this type of dementia.

What symptoms are usually present?

- Presents with sudden changes, stepwise progression
- Often the consequence of other conditions like diabetes or heart disease

- Damage is related to blood supply/not primary brain disease: treatments can plateau
- Unique to the individual (blood/swelling/recovery)
- May bounce back and/or have very bad days
- Judgment and behavior 'not the same'
- Spotty loss, inconsistent (memory, mobility)
- Emotional and energetic shifts

LEWY BODY DEMENTIA

Lewy body dementia is a form of dementia that occurs because of abnormal deposits of a protein inside the brain's nerve cells. These deposits are called "Lewy bodies," after the scientist who first described them. The deposits interrupt the brain's messages. Lewy body dementia usually affects the areas of the brain that involve thinking and movement. Hallucinations are a frequent symptom. Why or how Lewy bodies form is unknown. Lewy body dementia can occur by itself, or together with Alzheimer's disease or Parkinson's. It accounts for 5-15% of all dementias. When I personally picture these, I picture gummy bears stationed around the brain tissues, not letting the brain do its job.

What symptoms are usually present?

- Movement problems, will fall hard and often
- Visual hallucinations including animals, children, people
- Fine motor problems, typically related to the hands or swallowing
- Episodes of rigidity and/or syncope (temporary loss of consciousness)

- May have history of nightmares or insomnia
- Usually includes delusional thinking
- Fluctuations in ability/abilities can come and go
- Drug responses can be extreme and strange
  - Can become toxic and result in the inability to move or in death
  - May have OPPOSITE and atypical reaction

FRONTO-TEMPORAL DEMENTIA

Frontal-temporal dementia (also called Pick's Disease) tends to occur at a younger age than Alzheimer's disease and can affect both men and women. The average length of the disease can vary. This type of dementia resembles Alzheimer's disease in that it also involves a progressive degeneration of brain cells that is irreversible. With this form of dementia, a person may have symptoms such as sudden onset of memory loss, behavior changes, or difficulties with speech and movement. Unlike Alzheimer's disease, which generally affects most areas of the brain, frontal-temporal dementia is an umbrella term for a group of rare disorders that primarily affect the frontal and temporal lobes of the brain – the areas generally associated with personality and behavior, as well as speech and our filter for what is acceptable behavior. In frontal-temporal dementia, the changes in the brain affect the person's ability to function. Personality changes are an early symptom. Hallucinations are also common. Researchers estimate that approximately two to five percent of all dementia cases are frontal-temporal dementia.

What symptoms are usually present?

- Many types, typically younger onset
- **"Frontal"** includes loss of impulse and behavior control (typically this dementia doesn't present with memory issues)
- Will say unexpected, rude, mean, or odd things to others
- Has no ability to filter thought processes
- Dis-inhibited in behavior around food, drink, sex, emotions, or actions
- May include OCD (obsessive compulsive disorder type behaviors)
- Hyper-orality – putting everything in the mouth
- **"Temporal"** includes loss of language (speech and/or comprehension)
- Unable to word find, vague descriptions
- Comprehension limited, unable to understand, sound fluent – nonsense words

Our risk factors for each type are varied, but these risks all increase with age. But we don't have to freak out. We can understand what we may be faced with. All these types of brain diseases are just that, a disease. They are no more "normal aging" than cancer, or heart disease. Every disease has a progression and common patterns. Our challenge, should we develop a dementia, will be how to best cope with it before our thinking unravels, so we had better understand as much as possible and make a plan - just in case we forget.

CHAPTER 3

Challenges

Psalm 136:23
*He remembered us in our low estate. His love endures
forever.*

In other words, He remembers us when we are the
most difficult or helpless. His love endures forever.

Understanding some Challenges of Dementia

The challenges and obstacles brought on by this disease
are not insurmountable. But the dementia journey
can bring many trials that must be managed in order to
provide the smoothest voyage. Sufferers can be tossed
about on waves of loss and change. This journey is like
setting out for our end point on a sailboat in the ocean.
We don't get to choose to go first class on the fastest jet. It
is a journey – and it can be a very long journey. We, and

our loved ones must adjust the sails for each change and loss. Being prepared for possibilities and understanding why certain challenges occur as the brain malfunctions is essential to building a plan to navigate the waters of dementia. Preparing all the passengers in our sailboat for any rough waters by checking the weather – buy actively understanding the probable course of the disease – and adjusting the course to try to avoid storms. Another essential element to this boat analogy is the fact that all of our sailboats are different. No one has this disease in the same way. The Alzheimer's Association and other dementia organizations are fond of pointing out "if you meet one person with Alzheimer's, you've met <u>one</u> person with Alzheimer's."

The person with the disease needs help. They are still who they are, but now they are different. Their loved ones have to try to figure out how to help them to maximize the parts of their brains that still work… while they are still working. It may help to think of the disease as going backward in human development. When a baby is born it must be fed and changed. The baby cannot talk and communicates needs through behavior – crying, banging on things, or other behaviors designed to get attention. They throw food on the floor to indicate they are done eating. They fall down a lot when they are learning to walk because their brains are learning coordination and balance. They use their fingers to eat because they can't yet get the hang of using a spoon. They talk and they don't make sense. They get upset when we don't understand what they are saying. Everyone is familiar with how a baby communicates, and through the process they learn to grow and evolve. They eventually learn how to feed themselves with their fingers, then a spoon, walk, talk, and go potty by themselves.

One of the things that makes the journey through dementia so difficult is it also requires learning how to deal with losses that seem very basic. As most people journey through this disease process, it is the opposite of the baby's development, often called retro-genesis. A person may become incontinent; they may have difficulty talking or finding the words they need to communicate or talk gibberish; they may need to eat with their fingers, or drop food out of their mouths, they might fall down a lot; and they will need more and more care until they become totally dependent on a caregiver. The disease can rob the dementia sufferer of their "adultness", but they are still worthy of respect and dignity. They are adults and should always be treated as such. Every person suffering from this disease has a wonderful past. They have stories of success, love, creativeness, spiritual depth, and richness of a life lived. They – You – may have been a CEO, a teacher, a pastor, a sales person, or a NASA engineer, and now this disease is robbing them (or you) of basic abilities. I know I don't want any of the people who may care for me to talk to me like I'm a baby, and negate all the significance of who I am and what I've experienced.

It is interesting to note, brain scans done of a person with late stage Alzheimer's and an eighteen-month-old child are very similar in terms of the parts of the brain that "light up" (circled in white) or are working.

Positron Emission Tomography (PET) Scan
Alzheimer's Disease Progression Vs. Normal Brains

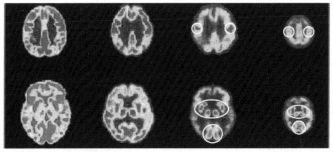

Normal   Early Alzheimer's   Late Alzheimer's   18-Month-Old Child
G. Small, UCLA School of Medicine

So this interpretation of dementia as human development in reverse, retro-genesis, although simplistic, seems accurate. The person suffering with dementia needs to know who will speak up for them when they can no longer speak for themselves. A developing child can rely on his parents to speak for them; parents who are with them 24 hours a day, meeting all their needs. Mommy can interpret a fussy cry from a cry of pain. Who will speak for you, and interpret your behavior – in case you forget?

If I get dementia, chances are my children will be making decisions for me. There will be lots of things they don't know about me because they haven't lived with me for a very long time, nor did they know me when I was a child. So I need to answer some questions about myself so that they can know me inside. How I think. What matters to me. What makes me comfortable and uncomfortable. Long-term memories and more recent routines will be important. It is important that a caregiver knows as much as possible about the history, background (including childhood), and personality type of the dementia sufferer. It will be easier to interpret any behavior as communication based on knowledge of who they were before the disease.

Jolene Brakey's book *Creating Moments of Joy (page 20)* contains a story of a man in his eighties suffering from dementia. He would walk around his memory care neighborhood saying "horse" over and over again. None of the caregivers could figure out why, or what to do for him. Finally, a family member remembered that when he was in his twenties (sixty years earlier) he had worked with horses for a living. They got a saddle and bridle for him and he spent many happy hours cleaning and caring for them.

Challenges can be met when we know a person's history This story illustrates that we need access to a person's whole history in order to figure out what they are communicating by behaviors. The richness of the life they've lived can bring depth and meaning and joy to the twilight of life. We can meet the challenge of this disease.

CHAPTER 4

Common Behaviors and What You Can Do

Deuteronomy 31:6
Be strong and courageous. Do not be afraid or terrified because of them, for the Lord your God goes with you; he will never leave you nor forsake you.

He is always with us – no matter what.

Common Behaviors

All behavior is a form of communication.
Five common behaviors associated with Alzheimer's disease are:

- Angry Outbursts and Physical Aggression
- Hand-wringing, Pacing and Rocking
- Accusing Loved Ones of Wrongdoing and Hallucinating
- Repeating Stories and Leaving the House Unassisted
- Sleep Problems and Sun Downing

Dementia turns our world upside down. Our natural response is to see someone as difficult. But the truth is; these behaviors are caused by the disease.

The first thing that must be done is to try to understand what is being communicated. Did something happen to cause the behavior? Imagine having to go to the bathroom, but not being able to find it. Are they experiencing any pain? Imagine your back hurts from compression fractures, but you aren't able to voice that. You just know you can't get comfortable. Are their needs being met? Are they hungry, thirsty, or have to use the bathroom? Can we change anything in the environment that might change the behavior (i.e. make it quieter or take the person outside)? Can you change your reaction? Try another approach? **Tip: Ask questions.**

If we realize that they are trying to communicate, it is easier to deal with behaviors we don't understand. If we try to understand the world from their perspective we may begin to understand their behaviors. Remember, their brains don't work, or they wouldn't act this way. When interacting with someone exhibiting challenging behaviors, always communicate you are on their side and they are right. Be in their corner. Validate their feelings. Their perception of the world is their reality. They can't help it, <u>but we can.</u> It is never okay to argue with someone with dementia. You will never win. If they saw things the way you do, there would be no need to argue. Their brains are not correctly interpreting the situation around them. So we, who can think correctly, must adapt.

I had some dental work done and was visiting my Mom and Dad, and my brother was there too. Now, Dad had dentures all my life, but he did not have them when he was a paratrooper in the Korean War. As we were discussing my teeth, Dad wanted to be a part of the conversation and said; "Did I tell you about the time I lost my teeth on a jump?" Both Mom and my brother wanted to correct him and remind him he didn't have dentures then, but he slammed his hand on the table and said; "*%&* I know what happened!" I drew close to him and looked him in the face, and said; "what'd you do Dad?" He said; " I caught them on my boot flipped them up and put them back in my mouth!" We all laughed with him. (My Dad was such a tough guy he'd put John Wayne to shame!) **Tip: Never argue.**

I knew a gentleman in a care home. His name was Joe. He was fun loving, with a great sense of humor, and enjoyed attention. Joe had been in the Air Force. He was proud of his service, and got positive affirmation for it. I'm not sure what his rank was, but toward the end of his dementia journey he would often say, "The General salutes you," in a very loud voice. He was never a General, but we treated him like he was. That was his perception, so we adapted. We didn't argue. Understanding behaviors is often easier if we knew the person before the disease, or at least have an understanding of their values and personality type.

Another woman I cared for, Claire, was from Greece and had lewy body dementia. She would "see" a little boy in her room very often in the afternoons. Sometimes she would start yelling at him in greek, or she would come out to find me and say in a very annoyed voice, "He's in there again." We would walk together back to her room where I would scold the little boy and shoo him out of her room telling him to find his mommy. That was her perceived reality, I just had to enter it and not argue. Telling her there was no little boy in her room would have greatly reduced her trust in me and accomplished nothing.

This technique for assisting them with coping with behaviors or their misinterpretation of reality is what I call *therapeutic lying.* It is entering their perceived reality and making statements that help them cope. **Tip: enter their "reality".**

For instance, Elizabeth would succumb to *sun downing* (late day confusion and agitation) near the end of the day and cry - wail really - for her husband Ray, who was supposed to pick her up. He had been dead for many years. She would wheel herself up and down the halls in her wheel chair yelling, "Ray!" It was very disturbing to others and it was hard to see her in such real distress. I decided to enter her reality and was able to tell her that I spoke to her husband on the phone (a therapeutic lie), and Ray asked if she would stay and eat dinner with us because he was going to be late. She was then much more agreeable to take her place at the table. This made sense to her in her reality.

One day Elaine, who I helped care for, wanted to talk to her son who had died a number of years ago. She was smashing her walker into the door and screaming that she had to get out of here and talk to her son. Everyone around her was getting upset because she was so upset.

She wouldn't believe me when I told her he was at work (a therapeutic lie) and insisted I get him on the phone from his job. She was becoming more aggressive and loud and began to use curse words. Finally, I was able to get another staff member to pretend to be her son on the phone, and she was assured that he was okay and would see her later. She was reassured and became compliant and happy and soon forgot that she had been upset.

Is there a "*therapeutic lie*" that would give **you** comfort in most situations where you might experience anxiety if you end up with dementia? It might be important to think about what your important relationships are and if you have any fears regarding them.

Redirection is a common technique in dealing with behaviors we don't know how to interpret. Refocusing a person's attention on something positive or safe. For example, if I know a person with dementia loves chocolate, then, when she becomes aggressive, or anxious, I can bring out a bar of chocolate (redirect her attention) and have it be "our little secret" that we are sharing the chocolate. I definitely believe in chocolate therapy! If someone who has had a deep faith life becomes upset or focused on a behavior that could be challenging, I may try singing a hymn, or saying the Lord's prayer with them. Activities involving one's faith are often comforting and calming. (I do know many people were taught to "behave" in church, so it can trigger good behavior!) **Tip: Know what they love!**

What do you love? What might be an effective bribe for **you** if you needed one?

"I want to go home!" is a phrase we often hear. No matter how *home-like* a care home is - it is not home to a dementia sufferer. The best way to redirect their attention and keep the behavior from escalating is to ask them about their home. "Sounds like you're missing home, tell me about it." This inquiry will bring up descriptions of the place or people in the home, so you can discover *when* the person is remembering. If they speak about their parents, they are likely thinking of their childhood home and the feelings of safety, security, and belonging that go with that memory. You can then interpret if they are feeling insecure, tired, or lonely and work to correct those feelings by affirming and validating them while they recall these feelings. **Tip: Ask questions to determine how to redirect.**

What about your home (childhood, young adult, & older adult) makes **you** love it? Why do you like your homes?

Music can make miracles. It creates mood as well as makes connections with pleasant memories. Wherever God put music in our brains it stays there, so if I know she sang in her church choir, I may be able to walk along with her in her wandering and sing Amazing Grace as we go. Soon her demeanor and anxious wandering can give way to a nice feeling of worship or remembering a feeling of belonging. I do find that most people interpret "church music" with being in church , so if behaviors have not escalated too much, a few hymns on the CD player will produce a fairly peaceful atmosphere.

I have great memories of all Johnny Cash music. I associate it with my Dad and his family. I usually know most of the words to Johnny Cash's top hits and they create a pleasant feeling of history and the security I always felt with my Dad.

Tip: Have several genres of music available.

What kind of music makes **you** happy? What kind makes you calm? What music reminds you of being in love?

Dementia changes people in ways that cannot be easily understood. It can be especially frustrating to caregivers who are just trying to provide for their basic activities of daily living. Bathing, for example, can become a real challenge. Do they have a need for modesty in everything? Can we cover areas that are not being washed and let them help to wash their private parts? Remember their brains are not interpreting the environment or our actions in the way we intend them.

I worked with a resident who had a brilliant mind. She had been a chemist and university professor. When she retired from teaching she had a cabin on a lake and she used to swim in the lake and generally commune with nature. She never married and considered herself an independent strong woman who was greatly respected in the scientific community. She had long greying hair and was refusing to bathe or have her hair washed. Her hair was becoming matted and unruly. The more the caregivers encouraged her to let them help her bathe, the more she resisted. I asked if I could try to help her and the caregivers were more than happy to let me give it a try. I prepared the facility bathroom with some classical music on CD, got wine and a wine glass with some fragrant bubble bath for the walk-in tub, then I spent about thirty minutes talking with her about how hard she worked throughout her life and validated her by praising her example of independence and strength. I then suggested that she deserved a relaxing bubble bath and that I had some special attendants ready to assist her. We had the lights turned down and the music playing with the bath running with bubbles. I met her with the wine bottle and glass and she grinned and said, "I believe I will." As an independent woman, when it was her idea, and she "deserved" it, she happily bathed and the staff was able to use this procedure (or a form of it) the next time she needed to bathe. If she had written down ways she liked to relax when she was younger, I bet a bubble bath would have been on her list. I didn't know, but I tried to guess based on the little information I had about who she was. **Tip: Know about past bathing habits and recreate if possible.**

What do **you** like about being clean? What bathing memories do you have that you might like to remember?

All of these coping strategies work much better when we know the person and have a good understanding of their personality before they developed dementia. If we know them, we have a much better chance of giving them good moments each day. Even if they don't remember the next day! If we have a history of who they are and what has been important to them throughout their lifetime it is easier to enter into their reality in a way that comforts and brings significance and value to them.

A person's history can provide rich insights into triggers that may manifest as difficult behaviors that must be navigated in someone's dementia journey. What part of your history might be important to know related to basic care giving? Did you hate the dentist? If someone tries to brush your teeth, might you think of unpleasant dental visits? Did you read on the toilet? What did you read? How do you like to relax? These are good things to know about yourself, and write down *in case you forget.*

CHAPTER 5

End Stages

1 Chronicles 16:15
"He remembers his covenant forever, the promise he made, for a thousand generations."

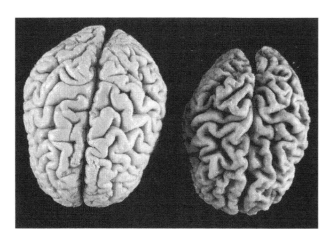

Normal Brain   **Alzheimer's Brain**
(brains of same gender and same age)

Of course, this terrible disease only progresses. It marches on, stealing pieces of our loved ones by inches at a time, until at last they are only able to respond minimally. People withdraw into themselves and may only allow glimpses of themselves and who they were. The five senses become the only ways they perceive the world around them. The senses themselves are often also impaired. The eyesight may be poor, they may be hard of hearing, and they may lose much of their fine motor perception skills. The ability to form words declines, as does the ability to string them together meaningfully. The goal of caregivers becomes providing as many positive sensory experiences as possible.

Sensory Stimulation is a must in later stages of any dementia. Again, if we know the person suffering from a dementia and their background well, we can be much more successful and impactful to provide a more positive quality of life!

Imagine being bedridden and unable to speak. Locked in a prison of this disease, your life is reduced to a bed in a room. Imagine you have always loved the old country music of Johnny Cash and Hank Williams, and have great life experiences with this type of music as background. However, because some caregiver read somewhere that classical music is good for the human brain, you are spending hours of your days surrounded by the notes of some symphony. What you wouldn't give to hear the *Orange Blossom Special* or *Hey Good Lookin'*. These songs that remind you of who you are and how you baled hay with your brothers. Many people associate certain songs with certain times of their lives. When disease robs us of the ability to create our own experiences, we will rely on our five senses for stimulation. We need to provide caregivers with a map of the sensory stimulation we've enjoyed.

Roy was in the end stages of his disease. He was nonverbal. Hadn't uttered a word for at least a year. Most of his joints were contracted and he was confined to his wheel chair. One afternoon we had a hymn sing with many old and familiar songs. Everyone was singing *Amazing Grace,* and I looked up at Roy. He was singing every word with tears streaming down his face. Somewhere deep inside, Roy was alive again and responding.

So music is a great idea - the <u>right</u> music makes the difference. All our senses can trigger past experience memories. There is a non-profit organization called Music & Memory[1] that has an amazing program that puts music from a person's era and preferences on a personal iPod with head phones to deliver the music effectively even if hearing may be somewhat impaired. They have some great information of the difference music can make in the quality of life for a person in the latter stages of this disease. Please look this up on the internet and you will see for yourself the joy that can be provided.

Think about the music of your life, special songs or eras of music that were the background to your memories… Songs and music create strong connections to your history.

Tip: Know what music genre makes connections for the person.

The sense of smell varies in its effectiveness in different people, but all of us can associate familiar smells with positive experiences. The smell of warm pumpkin pie and evergreen trees can produce happy memories of past holidays. The scent of gardenias often remind older women of corsages they got at dances in their younger years. Most people love the smell of hot coffee, or popcorn, or cinnamon. Just imagine a good memory and think of the aroma associated with it. Caregivers can hold scented wax cube under a nose to smell, or use a wax warmer or essential oil diffuser to engage the sense of smell. There is a lot of information about the use of essential oils and aroma therapy and healing touch with oils available to enhance the quality of life of dementia sufferers.

Senses can be combined as well. The scent of evergreen and Christmas carols are an obvious example of a good combo, add the scents of pumpkin pie or peppermint stick and you have a great sensory start to a positive experience and creating a memory of Christmas.

Many people in late stages of dementia respond with smiles and other warm facial expressions when receiving a hand massage with a pleasantly scented warm lotion or essential oils. Manicures, massages, going to the beauty salon, or a nice head massage all feel good. The feeling of touch is very powerful. Having someone brush your hair gently, give you a hug with their face touching yours, or simply hold your hand while listening to music, can make a connection that brings a welcome sense of belonging.

Pictures are very important as well. Even if a person rarely opens their eyes anymore, if they see a picture of their parents as they looked when they were "mommy and daddy" it can create a feeling of security and comfort.

If a caregiver is wise and wants to create a complete sensory experience they will choose a memory or common experience and provide five sensory items. For example, we might choose to remember babies for a woman who had children, babysat younger siblings, or liked babies as a child. Baby powder and baby lotion could provide olfactory stimulation, pictures of babies or a life like baby doll to hold, a CD or singing familiar lullabies together, and perhaps a drink of milk are all ways to bring that person a more complete baby experience. We could do the same with other themes such as a summer theme or a Christmas theme. **Tip: recreate a positive memory experience by using and stimulating each of the five senses.**

The point is, even at the end stages of the disease positive experiences can be enjoyed and made more positive if we are familiar with who a person is and what brings pleasure for them.

CHAPTER 6

Care Options

Isaiah 49:15-16
"Can a mother forget the baby at her breast and have no compassion on the child she has borne? Though she may forget, I will not forget you! See, I have engraved you on the palms of my hands…"

"What should we do?" Friends who find themselves with a parent diagnosed with dementia often turn to me when they find out what I do for a living. They want to find out what their options are. Traveling the dementia journey can be complicated and long. Families don't know what to expect or what their choices might be. Family dynamics also play a huge part in how this change in the norm is dealt with.

One daughter who lives close to her Mom and visits with her everyday expressed her frustration and fear. "I try to tell my brother three states away that I think Mom needs to be somewhere safer than the family home. I'm afraid her memory is so bad that she may burn the place down. I usually bring her dinner, but what if she decides to bake cookies or something?" It is easy to understand her fears. "My brother calls her and talks to her on the phone for five minutes a week and then when we talk about Mom he says, 'She seems fine to me. I think you are blowing things out of proportion.' I wish I could move her in with us or we move in with her, but it just isn't possible. What am I supposed to do?" This is just one version of many families who find themselves dealing with a loved one with dementia.

There are many care options along the journey should one be diagnosed with a dementia. Of course, part of the consideration may be additional health concerns combined with the dementia. If medical problems such as congestive heart failure or other heart disease, cancer, chronic obstructive pulmonary disease or other respiratory disease, or a fractured hip occur, the dementia journey can become more complicated. Each individual needs to find individualized solutions to what they are facing.

HOME CARE

Home care is the most preferred. No one wants to leave the home in which they are comfortable and familiar. Loved ones take on the role of caregiver most often. If we can maintain a familiar routine in familiar surroundings we can function more normally for a longer period of time even if we are faced with advancing dementia. Changes can exacerbate cognitive confusion for dementia sufferers.

Home Health agencies are often an important part of the team when keeping loved ones at home. Interviewing different agencies and individuals is a must. Helping the person with dementia feel comfortable with a "stranger" coming into the home to assist with bathing, medication administration or food preparation is very important. Be sure the caregiver has a good understanding of the disease process and its challenges.

ADULT DAY CARE

Adult Day Care is a great option for many. It is just what it sounds like. The day care provides a structured environment with many quality of life aspects as well as a good deal of the physical care - if needed. These organizations provide activity programs designed for shorter attention spans, places to pace/wander, and medical oversight to administer medications as prescribed. There may be limitations as to how much physical assistance is needed. This option can mimic the years spent "going to work" and can allow for family members to continue their own careers, while making sure loved ones are in a secure situation.

MEMORY CARE

A Memory Care Community is a safe long-term option where the care community meets all the physical needs and plans a quality of life activity program to fill days with positive experiences. Often when a loved one is worn out from caring for someone at home they find a Memory Care home to facilitate the hardest part of the physical care and then they can continue to enjoy their time visiting their loved one without the exhaustion of being the primary care giver. A word of caution and reality, they will be receiving care in a safe environment, but they will also be living with others suffering with dementia, so their day-to-day relationships and interactions will be with other sufferers who are not always responsible for their actions because of their disease.

HOSPICE CARE

Finally, Hospice Care provides many services and should not be viewed as simply the last step before death. Dementia is a terminal illness and hospice care can be a great option for dealing with the disease, as long as they qualify. People can be receiving hospice services, even during home care, and can receive hospice services for years. These services include assistance such as showers, dressing, and help with some nutritional issues as well as chaplain services and support for the family.

There are options out there and it is best to find all the assistance you can in choosing what you need. There are also businesses such as *A Place for Mom* (promoted by Joan Lundon on TV) that can help to find what you may be looking for. Keep in mind that facilities pay *A Place for Mom* to refer you to them, so you must do your own research as well.

And if you are making plans for yourself – *In Case You Forget* – check out places near one of your kids, and look at the star ratings the state board of health gives each care community. Write down what you think you would like to have available to you based on who you are. Do you want live music each week? Do you want a bath tub or are only showers okay? Do you want a private room or would sharing a room remind you of college?

CHAPTER 7

Universal Needs

Psalm 139:1-3
You have searched me, Lord,
 and you know me.
You know when I sit and when I rise;
you perceive my thoughts from afar.
You discern my going out and my lying down;
you are familiar with all my ways.

Quality of Life is defined as the standard of health, comfort, and happiness experienced by an individual. Before we can expand on what gives our lives quality we must first recognize the universal needs of every human; no matter their age.

- The need to belong.
- The need to love and be loved.

- The need to be useful.
- The need to be respected.
- The need to be responsible.
- The need to make choices.

These are the basics. I've included these universal needs so we can think about how they apply to us, and their influence on our quality of life. Remember, we are trying to have a plan in place about how we'd like to be cared for - *in case we forget.*

BELONGING

The need to belong starts when God gives us parents. A family unit. This then expands throughout our lives as we grow. We belong in a certain class from preschool through college. We belong to teams, we belong to organizations, as we age we might even belong to a senior center or to the Silver Sneakers groups at the Y. Belonging is basic. The need for belonging will remain even as we age. When evaluating our own belonging - during each decade of our lives - what memberships filled this need for belonging? What was belonging to your family like? Were you part of teams or organizations? How did they shape or influence you?

TO LOVED AND BE LOVED

The need to love and be loved also begins in our family unit. It is so basic that without it tiny babies often die due to what is called a *failure to thrive,* because they had no one to love them. Normally we learn to love and trust our parents as they love us. As we grow, we develop other relationships throughout life. Expressions of love come in many forms. We express our love emotionally, physically, and socially. Relationships often grow deeper and expand as family expands. We have a huge capacity to love given by our loving creator. Loving and being loved is a universal need. It's basic. What relationships have fulfilled this need to be loved in each decade of your life? Think back to all your significant relationships. Which have endured? How did each relationship impact you?

USEFULNESS

The need to be useful gives us a sense of value and pride in contributing to society. Our time and talents are ours to use to varying extents. Only when we actually give of ourselves can we feel useful and contribute to others or to a cause we value. As people age we still need to contribute, even after we retire from a paid profession. Much of the volunteer force in this country is made of retired individuals who still have a need to feel useful and contribute. They have a lot to give. Usefulness is basic. How have we contributed and felt we were useful throughout our lives? What did you do that made a difference for others and gave you a sense of pride and accomplishment in each stage of your life?

RESPECT

The need to be respected is an affirmation of our value. We demonstrate respect in many ways such as how we address those we love, those in authority over us, and those who hold societal roles of respect, such as the President.

Respect is a basic need that enforces who we are and how we are viewed by those in our sphere of influence. Being addressed as Sir, or being asked for your opinion by someone, are signs of this respect. Respect is basic. In what ways have we felt respected in our roles and relationships during our lives? In whose life have you had an impact? How? Was it different when you were younger?

RESPONSIBILITY

The need to be responsible is a lifelong process beginning with learning to take care of ourselves and our things. As my granddaughter is learning to use the potty her parents are very affirming of her learning this responsibility. Her parents are teaching her, as their parents taught them, how to respect others and share and put her toys away. Teaching her that she has responsibilities. As we grow we learn responsibility for ourselves as well as the health and safety of others. We show responsibility by using our talents and skills to earn a living, respecting rights and laws, and understanding and accepting consequences for our behaviors. Of course responsibility grows and changes with age, and nearing the latter stages of life we take the responsibility for what we want to happen when we are gone in the form of a will, or advance directives concerning health. Responsibility is basic. How have we shown our responsibilities as we have traveled through life? What was your most precious responsibility? How did it define you? Did you fail to fulfill any of your responsibilities? How did that affect you?

CHOICES

The need to make choices seems so obvious. Opportunities to choose our daily living, leisure experiences, and faith provide each of us with a sense of control, and independence. Making choices facilitates personal expressions, interests, preferences, direction and goals. These choices are often characterized by our clothes, housing, speech, education, titles in society, recreation and faith expressions. Making choices is basic. Some choices are big, impact our lives, and can change its course; some choices are as simple as what to have for supper, but choices often define our moments. What choices are part of who you are? Looking back do you always choose a certain color? Food? Political party? What choices have defined you? How? Why?

Maslow's Hierarchy of Needs pyramid is also know as Motivation Theory and was formed in the early 1940's. This one makes sense to me.

Maslow's Hierarchy of Needs

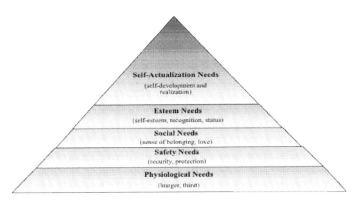

Self-Actualization Needs
(self-development and realization)

Esteem Needs
(self-esteem, recognition, status)

Social Needs
(sense of belonging, love)

Safety Needs
(security, protection)

Physiological Needs
(hunger, thirst)

There are other theories and ideas concerning human needs or stages of life and aging, regardless of which one we may subscribe to as the most accurate or as having the best science behind it, the truth is, humans have needs and these needs continue throughout our lives with adaptations as our bodies and minds may age.

These needs are universal. But we don't really think about them much. We just live life. As you age, which needs have become more important? Do you not really need a wide social circle as an older person, but you need to be addressed as "Doctor" or "Sir" because you have a high need for admiration and esteem? Take some time to think about what you will want those caring for you to know is important about you.

CHAPTER 8

Quality of Life

The quality of our lives is something we continually strive to improve upon, and deliberately enjoy. As most of us want to continue to have an enjoyable quality of life throughout our years, it makes sense to try to understand what we like, and are comfortable with in our lives. What is our personality type? Introvert? Extrovert? Nerd? Jock? What is it that makes life worth living for us? What standard of health, comfort, and happiness defines our quality of life?

Quality of Life; a standard of health, comfort, and happiness*; changes* due to our satisfaction and enjoyment during certain times in our lives. In the appendix of this book you will find a medical outcomes study of 116 core set of measurements of well-being. It is basically a survey to measure a person's satisfaction with their life. Take a look at it, do the survey yourself, and you will find that satisfaction can be found in all of the areas of human need, and satisfaction in one area can be affected by another.

A very specific example of satisfaction from my daughter's life, which will resonate with many women, is that she is currently pregnant with her second child, and her first is a toddler. She does not enjoy being pregnant. At all. The quality of her life is reduced due to the physical part of her life being uncomfortable. However most other areas of her life are very comfortable and enjoyable. Emotionally, spiritually, mentally, professionally, and even creatively she is satisfied. So the scales of a quality of life are tipped in a positive direction despite being physically uncomfortable.

People don't really talk too much about this when they are in their twenties, but when life brings more struggles, with health issues especially, quality of life becomes more important. We should always plan for a quality of life that brings joy NOW. To live in the moment and enjoy it - no matter the limitations. Taking time to evaluate the areas of our life that are most important to us and bring the greatest satisfaction can increase your awareness of all the areas that influence your sense of well-being. When we look ahead, we can be more specific about what we need.

In the long-term healthcare industry, Recreation Therapists and Activity Professionals are the staff members who are charged with concern for quality of life. The Centers for Medicaid and Medicare Services state in guideline F248 that "the facility must provide an ongoing program of activities designed to meet, in accordance with the comprehensive assessments the individual interests and needs of its residents."

The majority of staff in care facilities are clinical/medical personnel. I have worked as a Recreation Therapist for twenty-five years. This is a big job, and if I am unable to ascertain values, talents, and preferences of a person, especially due to advancing dementia, it is difficult to provide opportunities for optimum quality of life experiences. If the person isn't able to answer questions, it can help if family members can tell stories about their loved one. Our family history often reveals elements that hint at a person's quality of life values.

All life experiences can have positive and negative aspects, and all occur in *various domains* of experience. Physical, social, mental, and spiritual are some of those domains.

For example, my dad loved sports. I'm pretty sure he was good at everything he tried; football, basketball, golf, fishing, boxing, and even skydiving (of course, he called it Airborne, and it was during the Korean War). In the early/mid stage of his dementia journey, I had the opportunity to go parasailing with him in Hawaii. I knew it would remind him of his time in the Airborne, and I was ready to affirm his memories. If you've ever been parasailing, you know they strap you in harnesses, then let the parachute out and unwind the reel so you go up with the parachute. All you have to do is hang out and enjoy the ride and the view. It was a special time with my dad, until he started to pull on the lines holding the parachute, and I began to get a little motion sick. I was able to joke with him about it and he stopped trying to direct our landing so I didn't get sick, but I knew he was recalling actually parachuting and his physical domain memory was stimulated.

Experiences in the physical domain were a big part of his life. When his body could no longer actively participate, he adjusted his passions and coached, taught, watched, or talked about these activities. In this manner, he was able to continue the positive quality of life experiences in the physical domain. Keep in mind as well, that these experiences that Dad enjoyed were not purely physical, many were also social in nature. Teamwork and camaraderie (social domain) were part of what made these physical experiences, positive quality of life experiences, also.

Few people take time to examine what makes life experiences positive - ones we'd like to experience more often, or negative - those we'd like to avoid. This is how we can determine quality of life. More positive experiences than negative, give us a good quality of life. The most elementary examination is to break down the activity domains in which experiences occur. Next we will examine the domains in which our life occurs to further refine how to plan an *"in case I forget"* plan. There are <u>six basic activity domains</u>.

<u>PHYSICAL</u>

The physical domain includes the whole physical world, but mainly we are examining our own physicality. The things we enjoy that cause us to move and use our senses. Dancing, walking, jogging, swimming, yoga, sports - baseball, basketball, football, bowling, soccer, hockey, golf, boxing, volleyball, or, gardening, fishing, hunting, horseshoes, wood working, working on cars or other mechanics, swinging, gymnastics, cheerleading, biking, surfing, fencing, Tia Chi or other martial art are some areas to consider. Also included in this domain are the sensory things we've enjoyed. Our favorite foods, sexual intercourse, enjoyment of a bonfire, or involvement with nature are activities we enjoy on a physical sensory level.

Even breathing and being aware of how oxygen fuels our bodies, knowing how breathing deeply affects our alertness and awareness can bring physical pleasures and a positive physical experience.

Physical involvement in dementia can be vitally important. Positive responses to physical stimuli can make each day better. From a purely good for your health view point, *moving* at all stages of life is good for us. One behavior often exhibited by dementia sufferers is wandering. Walking, and walking seemingly pointlessly. However, if a caregiver can walk with a person and direct them to a positive physical activity such as sweeping the floor, hitting a balloon, or dancing to the music, much anxiety expressed through a wandering behavior can be abated.

When looking back over life, and contemplating the physical domain it will be wise to consider the whole picture of what has given our lives the quality we desire. Even if the physical domain is simply a memory of the quilt you snuggled in when you were reading the Hardy Boys mysteries. When evaluating our needs in the physical domain we need to think broadly and have good awareness of what has been important to us and why it contributes to our positive quality of life.

For example, I love the smell of cinnamon. As a young mother, I took some craft classes at a small town shop, and it always smelled like cinnamon. Now I associate the smell with creativity and hominess. I frequently melt wax cinnamon cubes in my home. It makes me happy.

What smells create positive memories and/or feelings for you?

EMOTIONAL

The emotional domain encompasses the things that engage our emotions. These are things we are passionate about or feel deeply. Emotional health can be enhanced through our expression of feelings. Discussion groups, music, bible studies, creative writing, art as expression, conversations and reminiscing, even watching a movie or reading a book that triggers emotions can foster positive feelings and are enjoyable when we are involved. Being recognized and valued for our contributions, feeling like we belong, being called by our preferred name, opportunities to share knowledge, abilities or skills are also an important part of emotional health. Interactions with pets or animals, small children or babies, making new friends, and being in nature have great emotional impact. Opportunities to laugh are important to emotional enjoyment, as are chances to volunteer and feeling valued and having a purpose.

Emotional interactions and emotional meanings for one suffering from dementia can be difficult to interpret; however, if opportunities to laugh, or reminisce through familiar venues are presented it can be a good day. Every time a caregiver says "good job" in response to something, she is creating a positive emotional bond and feeling of value with-in the dementia sufferer. For example, for someone who used to run a company, being asked his opinion about anything can create value and positive responses for that person. Understanding our emotional triggers and responses are important.

We often think of emotions as simply either negative or positive. We like something or we don't. Something makes us feel good or it doesn't. But evaluating our emotional domain is much broader and requires us to be fairly self aware when reviewing our own needs in this area.

Understanding your personality type and how God wired you can give one insight into understanding how the emotional domain affects our quality of life. If we enjoy people and are extroverted, chances are we will seek out others even when we don't really know why. If we are introverted and prefer our own company, we may withdraw and isolate ourselves. Understanding how we typically respond emotionally to our world, we can create more positive experiences than negative. Reviewing experiences in our lives in terms of emotional impact will help us evaluate the significance of a memory and the possibility of it "sticking" should we ever develop dementia.

Since I moved so often while growing up I have learned to "put myself out there" in a semi-extroverted way. I can have fun and make friends in new situations, but I much prefer quiet intimate conversations or being alone with a book to re-energize and re-charge. It will be important to know how I felt emotionally about being the "new kid" so often to create a positive experience for me should I develop dementia.

SPIRITUAL

The spiritual domain is important because it holds our belief systems. It defines us as having a spirit and how our spirit responds to God. Our faith lives usually have their roots in childhood. Often tied with our family traditions and moral upbringing. Most adults have an awareness of their spiritual beliefs, but it can be something that is often ignored until one deals with mortality in some way. Often it is a death in the family or a serious medical issue that brings this to the forefront of our thoughts.

Those who are dealing with dementia can respond to spiritual programs and interactions with surprising depth and insights. Even when they cannot form complete sentences they will respond reverently to holding hands and reciting The Lord's Prayer. I have had some very enlightening conversations after reading aloud a story from Guidepost magazine, and have seen the simple act of kneeling before a person who is crying (dealing with sun downing behaviors) holding her hands and asking if I can pray for her bring peace and moments of calm.

Spiritual health can be nourished individually or corporately. We may enjoy a personal devotion, prayer time, or bible reading routine. It may be during this time that we feel connected to God. It could be during a corporate worship service where our hearts and minds are focused and responding to God. The Lord's Prayer, or other familiar spiritual routine, may resonate in our spirit. Receiving communion or reciting the rosary may have significant importance to our inner self. Even being in nature and listening to the ocean or watching a sunset can move us spiritually. Music, either hymns or worship choruses, may draw us close to God.

Whatever your denomination or religion, it is important to understand your needs and responses in this domain and how they relate to your quality of life both now and in the future as you age. What impactful rituals or spiritual habits will be important should you develop dementia? When did you have a significant spiritual experience? Was it positive or negative?

It will be important to those caring for me should I develop dementia, to know that every morning I have a quiet time with God. As I've grown older I've added a cup of coffee or tea, but it always includes a time of journaling my prayers or insights from what I've read in the Bible or in a devotional book.

MENTAL

Dealing with a brain disease like a dementia, one would think the **mental/intellectual domain** of life would either be very important, or not important at all due to declining cognition. The answer is both, depending on what kind of mental involvement we have participated in all our lives. Our jobs certainly have a significant amount of mental investment and so do our leisure activities. Everything from reading a book or news report to playing cards and balancing our bank accounts require a certain amount of mental and intellectual investment. Problem-solving and decision-making are part of our everyday lives. Being able to think is a wonderful gift that we do not cherish until we are unable to think correctly. Games, puzzles, discussions, following cooking recipes, following a sewing or knitting pattern, committee work and volunteering, writing letters, ordering off a menu, keeping score, managing a budget, understanding and playing by established rules, even just talking on the phone all require a certain amount of intellectual stimulation. Life-long learning is also a great goal to have as we age. Everyone has thinking patterns and methods of obtaining a desired outcome for whatever the task at hand. As we evaluate how thinking has been significant in our lives and which memories required a great amount of mental input, we can determine ways in which we may desire to keep thinking or stimulating our cognition throughout the aging process. What mental activities will be important to us should we develop any cognitive impairment? Have you been a visual learner, kinetic learner, or auditory learner? Knowing this about yourself will allow you to continue to use mental capabilities, even as they fade.

I learn by watching and then doing. By reading and taking notes. In this YouTube era we can still learn so many things. I like to learn artistic things, and I love words, so I also enjoy word games like "*Catch Phrase*". This love of word games may be frustrating to me if I get dementia as most dementias cause word finding difficulties early on, so I may need an adaptation to an easy form of hangman perhaps.

CREATIVE

The creative/expressive domain often goes hand in hand with the emotional domain. Whether our creative drive expresses itself in knitting, painting, recycling, writing, decorating, dancing, crafts, drama, gardening, animal involvement, photography, singing, building, wood working, web design, blogging, cooking, or playing an instrument, we are creating something and are emotionally invested because it fills a need within us. We enjoy and feel satisfied when we are participating in this domain. Throughout our lives we may have experimented with creating a variety of beautiful significant things. Your chili recipe may be passed down through generations; your saxophone success in jazz band in high school is remembered whenever you listen to jazz or pick up an instrument.

The point is, while we may believe these past creative experiences to be of little significance currently, when we reflect on our lives, creative endeavors may have had more impact on us than we were aware. What creative experience would you like to relive or explore more deeply? Even if you say you are not creative, think about ways you like to express yourself or what kind of entertainment you enjoy. Movie? Plays? Concerts? Craft classes? Dance?

As a young teenager, I loved drawing and made several pencil drawings (carefully copied from a picture) for my dad's office. He always complimented my talent, and I remember his dad, my grandpa, teaching me how to sketch horses - which I also loved - by starting with the ear. If I have to deal with dementia, this may be a memory of significance if I try to draw anything. (It will probably be a horse - just tell me how beautiful it is!)

WORK: HOW YOU CAN CONTRIBUTE

Throughout our lives we must work to survive, and this is called the **working/contributing domain**. This has a large part to play in our identity. Especially for men. When men meet for the first time, many describe and define themselves by what they do. What is their significant job. Women also do this, but most always include significant relationships, such as describing themselves as a "working mother" rather than just by their profession. What we do for a living is always a way of contributing something that only you could do at that time, even if it is in the volunteer sector and there is no monetary compensation.

We all have a need to play our part. We can review our work history and each job we held to assess the significance each vocation had on who we are. Did we chose our job by gaining an education; or did it fall in our laps and was a perfect fit. These vocational paths are part of our story and could be noteworthy as we calculate what has given us value in our lives.

As we take time to review our work history, what are the meaningful parts of our careers? What are we most proud of? What caused the most stress or hurt?

I can tell you with a fair amount of certainty, after working in long-term care for more than twenty-five years, I will never want to play bingo if I can help it. I have called so many games of bingo and tried a variety of spins on bingo, such as Jingo, and pumpkin bingo, and other fun creative versions, but it has never stirred my heart or added any meaning to my life or my job. I have often joked, if I develop dementia and some well-meaning activity professional tries to make me play bingo, I may have some unpleasant behaviors as I try to communicate my dislike! Or perhaps I'll just take over! However, I believe I have created significant moments of enjoyment for many older adults, and have impacted their sunset years in positive ways, even if they didn't remember it the next day.

What about you? What significant element of your vocation is important to know and why? Did you work in different vocational areas or the same line of work for many years?

CREATING A NOW THAT MATTERS AND BRINGS JOY

Make NOW matter. Know yourself. Who you are *now*. Understand your motivations and personality. Ask God for insight into how He formed you. Make NOW matter, by paying attention. Everyday. Practice becoming who you are.

Consider starting a journal and noting highlights from each day, or make it a journal for daily prayers. Or make a gratitude diary, where you can write daily what you are thankful for. Focusing on the positive things of your life is always good for us. Like so many things in life, we put off forming new habits. We know we want to pray everyday - but we'll start…soon. Make NOW matter, so if you should become unable to speak for yourself, or express who you are, your long formed habits will have become such a part of who you are, they will still define you.

While we want to plan ahead, only God knows the plans He has for us. (Proverbs 16:9 & Jeremiah 29:11) He encourages us to plan ahead. I am suggesting we make NOW matter by forming habits that will be an ingrained part of who we are.

- If you want to be known as a grateful person, get into the habit of being thankful. Noticing all the blessings surrounding you and speaking thanks are wonderful characteristics to cultivate!
- If you know how important prayer is, get into the habit of praying about everything now. Then, if something should happen it will be your first response and not your last resort.
- If you love to laugh, laugh every day. Find something joyful or funny and laugh! Daily. Then you will be in the habit of seeing the lighter side of things.
- If you love deeply, express it…everyday. Be known by how you care. NOW.

One of the training exercises I've used is to ask team members to write on separate pieces of paper words (nouns) that describe them. Words such as: believer, person of faith, artist, reader, music lover, foodie, shopper, chef, Mom, daughter, wife, business owner, caretaker, scientist, Dad, brother, friend.

Then I ask them to choose three and crumple them up... The disease has taken this from them. Then after discussing what has been lost, I ask them to crumple up three more descriptors. The disease has taken that from them. Finally they have to crumple three more. This is very difficult, because the remaining words are closer to the core of who they are. Finally they're left with only one thing...

The first time I did this exercise, the facilitator just walked past the tables and took the papers. (they were folded in squares and neither she nor the participants could see them) So we just opened up what was left of us.

This is a powerful reminder to live deeply and fully in the present – everyday.

So instead of living for someday, make NOW matter. What/who we are now, will affect who we are in our eighties and nineties if we are fortunate to still be alive! Old age is a privilege denied to many.

CHAPTER 9

Three Steps

Psalm 102:18
Let this be written for a <u>future generation</u>,
that a people not yet created may praise the Lord.

So what should we do to be prepared for this disease? What should we do if we are worried we might succumb to this unraveling of who we are?

STEP ONE: FACE YOUR FEAR

No one wants to get sick. When most of us think about dying we all hope we will just quietly go to sleep. But we don't get to choose how our end will come. All through our lives we have made choices that might influence the possible outcome - but we never know.

If you are reading this book and have gotten this far - you probably have a fear of developing some kind of dementia. Maybe a relative had it. Maybe you're getting forgetful and you naturally jump to the worst conclusion. But if we are honest, we are afraid we may develop some kind of dementia and will lose our memories and lose who we are.

Just writing this makes me think of the scene in the 1991 movie *Hook*. Robin Williams stars as Peter Pan, but he is all grown up and unfamiliar to the Lost Boys. One of the boys looks intently at him and manipulates his face with his little hands, until finally pulling his face into a smile; he says, "Oh there you are Peter!"

We want our loved ones to be able to recognize us when we might be different. When they are losing us by inches to dementia, we are still there.

We won't let fear paralyze us. We can take steps to be sure we remain who we are. We just might be a different version of ourselves. So a contingency plan is in order. Covering of our bases.

What are <u>your</u> fears?

- Will you be a burden to your kids?
- Will you be unable to afford medical care should you need it long term?
- Will you lose your independence and be known by your disease instead of who you've been/are?
- Will the joys of life be taken? Hobbies, creativity, socialization and belonging?

Define your fear and make a plan. Let me help you.

IN CASE I FORGET

Jeremiah 29:11
For I know the plans I have for you," declares the Lord,
"plans to prosper you and not to harm you, plans to give
you hope and a future.

Plan for your fears. And trust God.
There are so many questions - only you can answer - *in case you forget.*

- How can you reduce the burden to your kids?
- If you don't have kids, who will be responsible for you? Make some decisions. Have some hard conversations - before you can't.
- Realistically look into what your options might be to pay for any needed long-term medical care. Educate yourself. Tell your loved ones what you discover.
- Take steps to assure you are not defined by your illnesses at the end of your life, but continue to be defined by who you are.

Life review can be very helpful in defining fears (and their origins), milestones, memories, and values of significance. Life review can also give a realistic determination of your personality.

For instance, do you like to be touched? My husband and I are very different in this area. He loves to have his back scratched, or to have feathery light touches on his arms or sides. He enjoys the goose bumps it gives him. I much prefer a back rub or firm strokes up and down my arms. This could be significant to know if you can no longer speak for yourself, or remember how to answer. So as you are completing a life review; also include your senses and personality type in the memory.

Answer a series of questions about your life and your personal notable memories. Evaluate how impactful or habitual each memory was. Look back by decades for organizational sake. I have included some of my memories as examples.

Answer the following questions thinking through childhood memories.

Describe the role your grandparents had in your childhood. Did they live nearby? Did you feel close? How did your parents talk about/to them?

_____

_____

_____

_____

Describe something you and your father did together:

_____

_____

_____

_____

Describe a way your parents influenced your spiritual beliefs:

_____

_____

_____

_____

Describe a time when you felt you were lucky:

_____

_____

_____

_____

What was a favorite saying of one of your parents?

_____

_____

_____

_____

For me: My dad had a great response when people asked him, "How are you?" He said, "I was okay, but I got over it." Now I like to respond this way at times!

My Mom rarely says a swear word so when encouraging her kids to figure something out she might say, "Get your poop in a group." Now I use this response at times, also.

What state or country did your father's family come from?

_____

_____

_____

_____

What is an unanswered question you would like to ask your parents? Your grandparents?

_____

_____

_____

_____

Recall a time you got in trouble at home:

_____

_____

_____

_____

Describe something your mother considered important:

_____

_____

_____

_____

Describe something your father considered important:

_____

_____

_____

_____

What is one way you and one of your parents are alike?

_____

_____

_____

_____

How did your parents meet?

_____

_____

_____

_____

Describe something you and you mother did together:

_____

_____

_____

_____

Describe your childhood relationships with your siblings. What did you do for fun? How did you bond together?

_____

_____

_____

_____

Tell about a special childhood friend. Are you still friends?

_____

_____

_____

_____

How did you discover your interests? Talents in art, music, athletics, academics?

_____

_____

_____

_____

Recall a time you got in trouble in school:

_____

_____

_____

_____

Describe something that made your father happy:

_____

_____

_____

_____

What is a game or song your family played or sang in the car?

_____

_____

_____

_____

For me: I grew up in six states, and no matter where we lived, we always took a trip to see my grandparents in North Dakota every summer. My mom was always trying to get us to look out the windows at the country. One summer there were herds of antelope and Mom was commenting on them. My little brother, maybe five or six at the time, asked "Do antelope come from cantaloupe?" and it became a funny family memory on all subsequent trips.

What are some ways you and your parents are alike?

_____

_____

_____

_____

How are your parents like their parents? How are they different?

_____

_____

_____

_____

Describe the role of money in your family of origin. Did you talk about it? Was it an issue? How did they save and spend? How has this influenced you positively or negatively?

_____

_____

_____

_____

Describe an event from your school days you will never forget:

_____

_____

_____

_____

For me: Some of my first school memories came in first and second grade. We were playing a chasing game in the gym, we called it boys chase the girls, and I was tripped, fell face first onto the gym floor and broke my new permanent front teeth off. I had lots of trips to the dentist after that. I also remember I got a coupon for ice cream after every visit!

Another dramatic memory was sharpening pencils at the pencil sharpener. I had my sharpened pencils in my right hand, turning the crank, and watching the pencil in my left hand get sharper - I jabbed the skin right next to my right eye with a sharpened pencil. After all the drama, my mom told me it was a beauty mark. I still have the blue/black mark.

Describe a favorite holiday tradition in your family. Think through each holiday (Sights, sounds, smells, feelings):

_____

_____

_____

_____

Describe the role of sports, band, math club, etc. in your life at this time:

_____

_____

_____

_____

Describe a favorite pet:

_____

_____

_____

_____

For me: We had BT - who my Dad named Broken Tail because he had a broken tail. He joked that he was a North American Indian dog. I went running with our dog BT after 10:00pm one summer night when I was 18, and he got sprayed by a skunk. I woke the whole family up when I brought him in to give him a bath in the basement laundry sink. Dad was not happy, but laughed anyway.

Any special relationships or memories associated with your extended family - such as cousins, aunts, uncles, grandparents?

_____

_____

_____

_____

For me: I have memories of a summer reunion of my dad's family and everyone watching the moon walk on the small black and white TV in my grandparents small living room.

I could share about memories of my cousins coming for Christmas when my uncle was deployed and my dad warning us to go to sleep and that he better not hear a "peep" out of us. Then my cousin Jimmy said "peep," and my dad cracked up.

I remember sleeping out in the back of my cousin Julie's station wagon while we shared with each other our experience of salvation and forming a relationship with Jesus.

Any regrets from childhood?

_____

_____

_____

_____

<u>Answer these questions while thinking back on your young adult years. Think in terms of your senses, too. Any smells or sounds (like music) associated with the experience?</u>

What was high school graduation like?

_____

_____

_____

_____

Favorite memories from college?

_____

_____

_____

For me: Involvement in the Fellowship of Christian Athletes at Purdue and meeting my husband.

How did you choose your profession/career? What are your favorite memories or how you changed and found what you liked?

_____

_____

_____

_____

What role did your vocation play at this time of life in defining you?

_____

_____

_____

_____

How did you meet your spouse? Describe it in as much detail as you can remember:

_____

_____

_____

_____

Describe your wedding:

_____

_____

_____

_____

Describe your first home:

_____

_____

_____

_____

Describe any moves to other locations:

_____

_____

_____

_____

For me: Prayers for my husband getting a job with the Fellowship of Christian Athletes and a song by an artist named Benny Hester, called _I Believe Something Good Is Gonna Happen Here_.

Did you have a pet?

_____

_____

_____

_____

For me: I had just had our first child, and we decided it would be a good idea to get a puppy to grow up with our son. We got a free puppy and named him Silly Nooper. We promised him a good home, but as I was caring for a new baby, this puppy chewed on EVERYTHING. I remember crying to my husband, "We promised this dog a good home, and I can't stand him right now!" I was crying real tears. "We have to bring him back." So we did. Years later when our third was a year old we got another puppy - a Cocker Spaniel that the kids named Gadget. We had her for fourteen years.

Describe how you started a family. Do you have memories around caring for babies, extended family involvement, celebrations, traditions?

_____

_____

_____

_____

Were your grandparents still a part of this time of life? If so, how were they important? Were your parents struggling with their aging? (If this is a fear for you, explore what your parents modeled and what you feel you are modeling to your children with your parents):

_____

_____

_____

_____

What did you learn from or about your parents while building your adult life?

_____

_____

_____

_____

How did you decide to do things differently than your parents? The same?

_____

_____

_____

_____

What are some strong memories - good or bad - you have about raising your family? What makes you happy to reflect on? What makes you sad?

_____

_____

_____

_____

What losses (grandparents, parents, pets, jobs, friends, marriage, or even a favorite car) did you experience during this time and how did they affect you? Did you grow or build walls?

_____

_____

_____

_____

What part did faith play in your life at this time? Is that significant looking back?

_____

_____

_____

_____

What role has your career choice had in your life? How important is this?

_____

_____

_____

_____

Children's teenage years can be challenging. What victories did you have? What difficulties?

_____

_____

_____

_____

How did your marriage change and grow in this time?

_____

_____

_____

_____

Any regrets from this time of life?

_____

_____

_____

_____

Answer these questions while thinking about your older adult years - 50 and above - remember to include sensory memories.

Describe memories of sending kids out into their own lives. Either college or first apartment/job etc.

_____

_____

_____

_____

Describe how you adjusted to an "empty nest":

_____

_____

_____

_____

What new talents or creative outlet have you discovered in this time?

_____

_____

_____

_____

What role did faith play at this time in life?

_____

_____

_____

_____

What role did your career play at this time?

_____

_____

_____

_____

Did you establish any new traditions? What were your holidays like?

_____

_____

_____

_____

Write about the birth of your grandchildren. Do you have memories about your own kids and your feelings of new life? Maybe you reflected on your parents as you became grandparents?

_____

_____

_____

_____

Describe how you feel about aging and the death of your parents? Any challenges? How did they affect you? What is your relationship with your siblings like? (Define your fears here):

_____

_____

_____

_____

Write about any job changes as you headed to retirement:

_____

_____

_____

_____

Describe any health issues:

_____

_____

_____

_____

<u>Know your Values</u>

Describe a possession you would like to keep if all else were lost:

_____

_____

_____

_____

Describe an occupation you think would be fascinating:

_____

_____

_____

_____

If you could do anything you wanted and cost wouldn't be a factor, what would you do?

_____

_____

_____

_____

What is a characteristic in others that you admire?

_____

_____

_____

_____

If you had more money what would you change about your life?

_____

_____

_____

_____

What is something you would do with your time if you didn't watch television?

_____

_____

_____

_____

Have you ever done a personality test? How would you describe your personality? (Remember to include your senses) Introvert? Extrovert? Leader? Follower? Artsy? Detailed? Loyal?

_____

_____

_____

_____

You completed a thoughtful life review by reading through and answering these questions. You have established some very clear memories with significance in your life. Some were fun to think back on and some were hard, but if you remembered them, especially if you recalled them in vivid details, they are part of who you are and they will always be part of who you are. Even if you forget the details or the names, the emotions, sensory elements, and resonance in your soul will remain.

Now what?

STEP TWO: WRITE IT DOWN

Write it all down in a format that your family or caregivers can understand.

- Buy a pretty journal and hand write all your memories and wishes.
- Type every answer and desire for *in case you forget* and put it on a flash drive for each child. (What a stocking stuffer!)
- Or just get a three ring binder and some notebook paper and start answering the life review questions.
- Even go old school and record the answers on a cassette tape.

Here are four formatting ideas for writing your memories and wishes.

1. In Quality of Life Domains:

Another way of writing down your wishes is to remember your significant experiences or feelings from your life review and pick out the ones you want to focus on. Express why or what part of the memory is deepest in your heart and makes you feel most like you. Think in terms of the activity domains – Physical, emotional, spiritual, mental, creative, work, and NOW. For instance:

Social Domain: I like playing games and enjoy recreational companionship. I like to meet new people during fun interactions of games I understand. *Note - I do not like bingo. :-)

<u>Emotional Domain:</u> I enjoy being by myself. I enjoy reading and entering into the story. Same for movies. I like people, especially in small doses. I enjoy learning and connecting with others. I'm mostly introverted, but can rise to the occasion and can speak in front of others in bible study or about something else I'm passionate about.

Other easy templates:

2. About Me:

An "about me" is a really easy way to capture your memories and desires, *in case you forget.* Here's an example of things you could write:

1. I like to be called _____. (Names are powerful. My husband was playing Santa recently and a friend and her small child approached. The little girl asked my husband if he (aka Santa) knew her name. When he told her her name she turned to her mom with eyes as big as saucers and said, "He knows my name!!" So write down the name your friends and loved ones call you. It will make you feel special.)
2. I grew up in:
3. Important people in my life include:
4. I used to live in:
5. I used to work as:
6. Previous life experiences include:
7. My current daily routines are:
8. My younger daily routine was:
9. My favorite places to visit are:
10. My favorite things to do include:

11. My favorite foods are:
12. I believe (types of activities) will always be important to me:
13. One thing I'm very proud of is:... because...
14. Sensory experiences I really enjoy are:
    A. Sight-
    B. Sound-
    C. Touch-
    D. Taste-
    E. Smells-

Remember to include all vivid memories associated with these questions.

3. As a Healthcare Goal:

In healthcare, each discipline has care plan goals for the patient. For example, a nursing care plan might read like this:

<u>Problem:</u> Patient has a diagnosis of COPD (chronic obstructive pulmonary disease - a chronic lung disease that makes breathing difficult).

<u>Goal:</u> Patient will maintain O2 blood saturation of 98% or higher.

<u>Approaches:</u>
Patient will receive breathing treatments as needed to maintain open airways and more effective breathing.
Patient will do deep breathing exercises daily to keep lung expanded to full capacity.

Patient will cease smoking to decrease risk of further lung damage.

Patient will receive O2 per nasal canola as needed when saturations fall below 95% to maintain optimal blood saturations.

Observe cognition or increased confusion as a sign of lower O2 saturations.

So, how can you write down your "plan of care" in case you develop a dementia?

Following the medical model the problem might be stated:

Problem: Patient has a diagnosis of (early, middle, late) stage dementia ___type.

Goal: *Name* will maintain enjoyable quality of life as evidenced by actively participating in activity or experiences that cause smiles or laughter. Specifically_____.

Approaches:

Name will participate in singing her favorite hymns as she has history of singing in church choir.

Name will participate in reminiscing about favorite holidays, especially Christmas by using sensory items of gingerbread, pine scents, and carols.

Etc…

Goal: *Name* will feel secure and safe and evidenced by calm demeanor.

Approaches:

Name will enjoy security during bible reading and prayer.

Name will become calm when instrumental hymns are played.

Name will continue familiar routine of reading the paper and drinking coffee each morning.

Etc…

4. Decades:

The last way you can easily write out your plan is by decades. Here's how:

As a young child (1-10) a significant memory is:

School age (10-20) memories include:

- Elementary
- Middle School
- High School

Young Adult (20-30) significant life events and people are:

Adult (30-40) important things about this time were:

Adult (40-50) The plans I was making with these people I love were:

Older Adult (50-60) The things I'm planning for retirement are:

Or make a template that makes sense to you.
You can be as in depth as you desire.
The main point is to <u>Write. It. Down.</u>

#

STEP THREE: SHARE IT

Think of this as an insurance plan. You are taking time to do all this "Just in Case" you are diagnosed with dementia of some sort. Step three might be the hardest for you, or it could be the most precious time.

You <u>must have a conversation</u> about this difficult topic.

If you are of a certain age, thinking about the future seems logical, but if your kids are young(ish), you might catch them off guard.

My parents, like many folks in their fifties or early sixties, decided to make their funeral arrangements and get everything paid for so it wouldn't be tough on us kids when they passed. I will never forget my mom calling one day. I wasn't prepared for this topic at all. I was in my thirties, and she called and said, "Dad and I are finishing up our funeral arrangements. Do you care if there's a body?" Really hit me out of left field. We went on to discuss it, but I must say I felt pretty awkward to begin a conversation with. "Do you care if there's a body?"

But, this is important. No one knows you like you know yourself. Even your spouse of fifty years may not know some impactful memory of your childhood. Good or bad. You have taken the time to write your history. Your story. Your important memories. Share them. Don't just put them with your advanced directives and hope someone will understand your wishes. Share this.

This could save you should you become a sufferer of dementia, from experiencing or re-experiencing unnecessary heartache, and could save your loved one from being unable to assist you in your dementia journey.

BEFORE YOU YOUR MEMORY UNRAVELS – YOU CAN HAVE A PLAN!

So this is how it might work - in case I forget - and have some form of dementia. Before my memory unravels, I wrote down all my vivid memories so my caregivers could know all about the "me" inside.

Imagine a dog visits the memory care home where I live. It's a black dog, and I start holding my nose. Because I have it written down, my caregiver, my daughter, or whoever has read or heard my stories, may say, "You had a black dog didn't you. Patty? You told me about a time you went running with your dog, and he got sprayed by a skunk. What was the dog's name?" If I can still talk I may finish the story, tell about how his name was BT, and I woke up the whole family when I took the dog to the laundry room sink for a bath. The memory will make me smile. My quality of life for that moment is very good and enjoyable. I am able to make others smile with my memory, and then I may also enjoy the black dog who is visiting as I remember BT.

However not everyone has happy dog memories. I knew a man who had been a postal mail carrier and was a veteran of WWII. His wife was able to tell me that he had had several dog bites during his time as a mail carrier and so was very afraid of dogs of any kind or size. Luckily his wife told me about it so I made sure he was never exposed to visiting dogs and never had to relive those bad memories.

I hope I don't ever get dementia of any kind but,

In Case I Forget,

I have a plan! And so can you!

Endnotes

1. https://musicandmemory.org/

2. https://www.rand.org/health/surveys_tools/mos.html

3. https://www.ncbi.nlm.nih.gov/pmc/articles/
   PMC2880929/

4. http://www.wai.wisc.edu/pdf/phystoolkit/
   screeningtools/Animal_Naming_form.pdf

Made in the USA
San Bernardino, CA
15 June 2020

73527096R00062